Legal Notice

How I Cured Chronic Pain and Digestive Problems: What REALLY Causes Back Pain, Joint Pain, Arthritis, Indigestion and RLS, and How to Get Rid of All Chronic Pain for Life - Fast, Easy, Cheap!

"Let my body go."

Table of Contents

You're in your mother's womb. You're suspended in the fluid, shoulders back, arms bent, legs curled and jammed up tight into the hip socket. This is the position your body's DNA is naturally programmed to accommodate, and in which your bones, muscles, nerves and joints are most comfortable. This is the position you need to return your bones.

I'm Chris Klein, premier case for chronic back and joint pain (aka arthritis) and a whole host of other health problems, most of which will be addressed in this unique e-book. Growing up I put unruly stress on my hip, spine, knees, and shoulder, thanks primarily to muscle imbalances in the hip. When I say muscle imbalances, really I mean weak muscles. There are a whole slew of muscles in the body that we rarely work hard, most of them attached to the hip and/or spine.

This really is the single greatest source for back, neck, and joint pain relief. This is the most comprehensive, clear cut guide you will find to ending problems you have been dealing with in your back, neck, and joints. I share it all - perfect postures and problem solving techniques. This guide is all about getting answers to the problems, not just masking the pain. You can mask all the pain you want, but that alone doesn't put a dent in the real problem.

Pain is actually helpful if you think about it. How would you know there was a problem in your body if it didn't give you signals to tell you so? If you didn't know your knee was deteriorating, you would keep using it and eventually wear it out to the point that it would need surgery to be repaired (if it could be repaired). So you don't want to "kill the messenger" so to speak, but rather find out what the messenger is hollering about.

Truth is, this book is like pure gold. I would have given anything, all I had even, to know a lot sooner in my life what you're about to find out. It's going to save you time, erase the pain a lot quicker than the average back pain sufferer and chiropractor patient, and slash wads of cash in medical bills you could rack up without this knowledge. No more wasting time, money, and pain. I did all the wasting for you.

You really can get 100% relief from all back, neck, and joint pain. You'll also learn the cause of chronic headaches/migraines, sinus pressure, and a whole host of uncomfortable sensations we feel in our bodies. You can do it! This book has your answers! You can get the relief you've been longing for - very soon!

This isn't some chintzy exercise or stretch manual, so as to sort of cover the problem or address half of it. This is finding the problem, putting it under a microscope, and getting rid of it - for good, for ever. No drugs, herbal therapies, surgeries, pads, creams, smelly ointments or the likes. I'm sure you're tired of all those ads, magazines, and health reports claiming to offer relief of your pain (I know I was). Yet rarely, if ever, will they tell you exactly what's causing the pain.

Now you can know, and not just get some relief from it. Now you can get the truth, fix the problem, and get bona fide relief of the pain. I laser-target the sources of your problems and shoot them with the right techniques. No more back pain, arthritis, headaches, etc.!

I'm not one of those doctors who *thinks* he knows it all or he knows what's good for you. This is coming from someone who experienced the pain and discomfort in the back, neck, and joints, and got the answers to the real problems. If you were a beginner baseball player, who would you rather have explain to you how to play the game right - someone with plenty of experience? Someone who went through the trials and errors and tweaked every technique and move until he perfected his game? Or from someone who just did a lot of research on baseball and occupied a seat in the front row of the ballpark? Someone like Barry Bonds, or Derek Jeter? Or your baseball-crazed uncle who's never stood behind the plate once? I'll take Bonds!

Take it from a Bonds of back, joint and neck pain; though I have something much more valuable than Barry Bonds could ever obtain. I have completed the puzzle that is back, joint, and neck pain (and chronic headaches, sinus pressure, etc.). I have put the pieces together. My pain and weakness is gone. Done. Boom. Sianara. See ya. Have a day! Never to return. The problems have been found and fixed. And I am not on any drug, pain reliever, heat pad...nothing! Just some good ol' knowledge about the right techniques to keep my spine, hip, and joints in balance and strong. It's all automatic for me too. Whenever I feel something get slightly uncomfortable, I just go and flex a muscle or two and it's all better. And my body - every day, all day - is saying "aaaah yeah." Some times I could just pass out I'm so comfortable and relaxed. I often do.

When implementing this program, keep in mind this very important thought: pay attention to detail. This is what made possible my full recovery from all the pain. It's also what has led me to keep the pain away and repel injury, forever. In fact, this whole book can be attributed to the attention I pay to detail; and to the way I guess, test, and revise things until I find what I'm looking for. I know what positions hurt my hip and joints, and what positions they love. If it hurts, don't do it. If it feels good, keep doing it. Keep these principles in mind, and you will find the answers to your specific problem(s). This will guide you to your answers. You will get complete recovery from your back and joint problems. Grind it out! Maintain an open mind! Believe!

You can start in on these techniques as soon as you want. Right when you find your problem and the answer later in this guide, you can start. Today even (if it's early enough).

The Basics

Your spine is a bunch of bones, known as vertebrae, stacked on top of each other to support your upper body. Surrounding and connecting these bones are ligaments, tendons, joints, discs, and muscles. Running through the spaces in between and through these bones and tissue are nerves. Nerves are not meant to be pressed on very hard. As I'm sure you know they're very, very sensitive. If any abnormal amount of pressure is put on the nerves, pain or discomfort is felt. This is, most of the time, why people undergo chronic pain. That's it, nerve interference. Abnormal amounts of pressure are being put on their very sensitive nerves. Misaligned vertebrae can put pressure on the nerves that run through them. This is a major source of pain and discomfort in the body, and on which most of this guide will focus. Numbness and strange, chronic pain or discomfort in the extremities can also be a result of this nerve pinching. These problems are what this guide is going to help you understand and overcome.

Sometimes people will just pull a muscle or ligament in their back, maybe from a lift, or accident. This will also cause pain because, obviously, nerves run through them. But this kind of damage is usually healed naturally by the body. This temporary pain is not the kind of pain this book about. Heat pads, some TLC, and nutrients will speed the healing process in these cases.

If you've ever seen a diagram of the spine, you'll notice it has natural curves to it. Putting enough force against these curves will cause the vertebrae to slip out of their natural alignment. When this happens, the space that the nerves had to run between the vertebrae suddenly gets taken away. Now, to some degree, depending on how far out of alignment the vertebrae fell, the nerves are being pinched. If you've ever heard of someone "pinching a nerve", this is what's going on. And they make it clear how painful it is. To some degree, you are experiencing this wherever your back, neck, or joints are hurting.

Now, what's causing the vertebrae to slip out of their natural alignment? This is the part the average doctor and chiropractor can't tell us. The foundation of the spine is the hip. As the hip goes, so goes the spine and other joints, I say. When the hip shifts out of its natural alignment, because of an overdeveloped muscle yanking on it, it will tilt the spine in an unnatural position. This shift can cause other bones and joints to shift as well, like the knees, or even the ankles - like a domino effect. This is the case every time, in my experience.

Ever played with a GI Joe action figure? I did when I was a kid. The hip on a GI Joe doll is remarkably like the human hip. The hip socket is held to the mid section by a small, tight rubber band. You can pull the legs down from the mid section on a GI Joe figure. Little did I know that was going to happen to me some day. That's what's going on in your bum hip, and what's causing your spine to tilt. Your hip is being pulled out of its socket, to some degree. The goal will be to suck your upper body and legs back into the hip socket by strengthening core muscles.

So, what causes a fluctuation in hip and joint alignment? Another concept foreign to some of the most well educated, well funded people on the planet.

The cause of hip displacement is a simple muscle imbalance. The source of most aches and pains in the body is a structural problem.

Your hip has 18 muscles attached to it. A lot for one joint, huh? A weakness, or imbalance, in any one of these muscles can cause problems to the hip bone, spine, and nervous, reproductive and/or digestive systems. A combination of two or more weak muscles can spell disaster to any of these systems. It's unlikely that just one or two muscles in your hip are underdeveloped. It's likely a combination of weak muscles letting the hip slide out of its alignment.

Unless you're ambidextrous (left and right handed), the primary core problem muscles are on the dominant side of your body. That was my problem - being heavily dominated by my right side (before I corrected the problem). If you're ambidextrous, the problem is likely just the muscles in the middle of your core.

The more developed muscles that we use regularly, every day, are yanking on your hip bone. The real problem is an imbalance between your leg and back muscles, and the weaker, neglected muscles in your core. Your leg and back muscles can actually work against and stretch out the muscles in your core. This will force the hip, spine, and other bones into unnatural positions, resulting in nerve interference (pain and discomfort). In my experience, this instability in the hip can affect any part of the spine – top to bottom – and even shoulders, knees, and ankles.

If you sort of walk a little funnier than you used to when you were very young, your hip is 'there'. It may not be terribly uncomfortable, for now, but letting it go will eventually cause some real discomfort. And if walking or running really hurts your hip area, you've probably been there a long time. Your hip is sort of coming unglued. We have work to do.

Another contributor to weaker muscles is constant poor posture. Sitting and sleeping positions can stretch out the more neglected muscles around your hip and spine. Office workers, musicians, or someone who has to be on their seat a lot during the day are prime victims of this problem. I had an old friend from high school (she was a musician and did manual labor in the family farm) who used to let us know clearly when it happened to her. My college and office work, combined with a lot of athletics and heavy weightlifting, set me up real well for it. All of our sitting, reclining and sleeping just destroy the posture.

The bulk of this guide is geared to uncovering and fixing the most common problem of all structural problems – hip and spine misalignment, and its effects. This book will address the most common underdeveloped and neglected muscle groups in your body. I will also touch on other common pesky structural problems in other joints.

The overdeveloped, problem areas around the hip are the hip abductors, hip adductors, hip flexors, thighs, and back muscles. The underdeveloped, weaker muscles being yanked on are the abdomen (6 pack), pelvis, and dominant side external oblique (if you're not ambidextrous). Combine these muscle imbalances with poor sitting and sleeping postures, and you stress out the hip joint virtually all day, every day.

The hip abductors are responsible for balancing when you walk, run or stand on one foot; and also for extending your leg out to the side.

The hip adductors are responsible for contracting your legs together and rotating them forward. This is a very bad motion, by the way. We utilize these adductor muscles constantly, while their antagonistic muscles – pelvis, abdomen, etc. – are rarely utilized, and even stretched out while sitting. The adductors are actually a set of 3 muscles.

The hip flexors are responsible for kicking the leg forward when you walk and run.

The thighs are responsible for extending the leg, of course. But there's a connective tissue on the side of the thigh responsible for balance as well – the iliotibial band, aka the IT band. For practical purposes, I will consider it part of the thigh from here on out.

I'm sure the back needs no explanation.

The abdomen and pelvis have strange motions. You'd think they were responsible for just pulling the upper body forward, but I've learned that they are responsible for pulling the hip bone up and back as well.

The external obliques are responsible for pulling the side of your hip bone up toward your arm pit. They appear to play a slight role in hip rotation.

These underdeveloped muscles actually serve a dual purpose. They all work in concert to slide the back of our hip bone up into its socket - along with the leg bones - neutralizing the stress from, and stretching out, our lower back and leg muscles. The result is perfect posture. You'll feel what I mean when you get done with the workouts at the end of this guide. This simultaneous slide of the hip and leg bones is the whole goal in correcting hip and spine related structural problems.

Bad Muscles:

Back
Hip adductors
Thighs
Hip flexors (Pectineus)
Glutes (butt) (it's true)

Good Muscles:

Abs
Pelvis
Dominant side oblique
Traps (Trapezius), rotator cuff, rear deltoid and triceps (for shoulder and neck issues)

I notice some athletes tend to have severe hip problems and end up with hip surgery. I can see how they would incur a muscle imbalance. Their adductors, abductors, flexors and thighs will get real tight from all that kicking forward and balancing. I once read in a strength and conditioning forum on some website about someone who was doing squat lifts one day and they felt something in their hip shift, and experienced some kind of problem ever since. That was a bone being pushed out of alignment and yanking on core muscles, all because of jacked up legs.

People who work their abs a lot might have overdeveloped adductors and flexors as well, after constantly squeezing them doing traditional ab workouts on a bench or floor. The hip flexors and adductors are already jacked up just from walking and running most of our lives. Most traditional ab workouts further tighten them. All this activity destroys posture.

Keeping the hip aligned can help you perform better, if you are an athlete. And it can even help you perform your ordinary, every day, routine tasks a whole lot smoother.

When you hear about people "throwing" their backs out or undergoing nasty sensations in the neck and back, it is the natural alignment of the vertebrae that has been effected. They wrecked their posture. The bones slip out of their place and pinch the nerves between them, due to weak muscles or an accident, or a combination of both. I once read an article about a dude who kept throwing his back out so badly that he would fall to the ground in agony - one time while standing at a urinal in a public bathroom! It went on to say that he benefited mightily from exercise because he had weak "core" muscles.

Not only will these misaligned vertebrae be pressing on your nerves, but, since they are out of their natural place, the muscles and connective tissue surrounding these vertebrae will be forced into unnatural, often times very uncomfortable positions. They will be forced to sort of make up for the lack of support the misaligned vertebrae are giving. This will soon result in fatigue and constant irritability in the muscles and tissue. If it's bad enough, muscle relaxers, drugs, and the likes will not be able to provide relief. The only way to get relief is to fix the problem. This is why I am in direct opposition to the medical and pharmaceutical communities regarding back and joint pain. They don't fix these problems, but rather try to ease symptoms. I'm no dummy. I'm going after the problem, and I will tell everyone the same. Every person who has even half-heartedly attempted my techniques has gotten relief. All who haven't attempted didn't. Fixing problems won't give me unwanted, unexpected side effects. Fix the alignment and everything around it - all the connective tissue - will heal back to normal.

The muscles around your hip and spine act much like support cords. They are to the spine what ropes tied to stakes in the ground are to a tent. Without ropes at the corners of a tent, it would sway and rock with the slightest breeze or tug. It would have the potential to get completely blown away in a strong wind. If the ropes are there and tied to the tent, but had some slack in them, the tent might bend. This is very similar to the relationship your muscles have with your bones. If your core muscles are loose, there isn't much stiffness there to neutralize the stronger muscles and keep the spine from shifting out of its natural alignment. Enough stress put on a hip and spine with loose core muscles will easily force the vertebrae out of alignment. The same goes for any other joint and its attached muscles.

Other Problems That Can Occur When Nerves in the Spine are Being Pinched.

In my case, in one spot, the sciatic nerve was being pinched. This is the big long nerve that runs through the leg - very important one. As a result, I lost a little feeling in my foot and my calf muscle seized up pretty good. I guess this is part of sciatica. It sort of felt like spasms in my calf but didn't hurt. It was really tense and uncomfortable. I would sort of squeeze on it, but it just seized up more when I did that. Hopefully you're getting a sense of how dangerous pinched nerves can become.

Now, since getting the bones in their proper alignment and learning how to keep them that way for good, performance in my legs is optimal and I get to completely feel my nice, plush carpet on my feet and toes.

A sure indicator of nerve interference is numbness in the extremities (toes, fingers, etc.). When nerves are pinched to the point where you lose feeling, you could be setting yourself up for serious problems, if you're not already there. If this is happening to you, you must find out what you're doing that is causing misalignments in your vertebrae and joints, and pushing them so far out of alignment that they're pressing on the nerves. You could be working a particular muscle group too hard, and not working its antagonistic muscle group enough, if at all. Maybe years of poor posture has pushed your vertebrae way out of alignment. It's very likely a combination of positions/motions. Think, and adjust accordingly.

More symptoms of nerve interference are: that tickling sensation in the inner ear, chronic dry eye, headaches, any strange or painful sensations in the head and sinuses; restless leg syndrome (you're laying in bed and your legs get the urge to move or get up), and other searing or shooting pains you may be experiencing. This is all nerve interference, a result of poor posture and a bum hip.

Baldness appears to be a structural problem as well. I found my hairline quit receding when I fixed my posture. At times when I get lazy and let my hip and posture suffer, and then work my abdomen real good, I feel a nice sensation in my scalp, like the nerves are beginning to fire again.

All these, and more, are symptoms of poor posture. The curves in your spine are getting pulled out of their natural position, anywhere from top to bottom, and your nerves are being pinched.

Arthritis

Earlier I mentioned arthritis. The real causes of arthritis are what you are about to learn, and have already learned, in some of the sections of this book. I know what it feels like. I have proven that muscle imbalances (one set of muscles being stronger than their antagonistic counterparts) and misalignments of the bones are those causes. By keeping a muscle group tense over time without countering the tension with the other group(s), the alignments of the vertebrae and joints stuck in the middle are pushed out of place. By further continuing this tension, cartilage begins to wear away and bones eventually begin to rub together. That is why one will experience crunching sounds and extreme pain under this debilitating condition - their bones are rubbing. And the "experts" are a little right when they recommend exercise for arthritis; they are addressing some of the problem. This exercise is why the pain can be eased up. Exercise can also trigger arthritis. The results of arthritis are joint inflammation and muscle stress. Arthritis puts much pressure on the structure of the muscles and connective tissue around the joint.

In joints outside the hip - whatever position your muscles have been flexing toward for so long, causing you pain - you will need to do an exercise that works the body part(s) in the opposite direction. I used to work in an appliance shop and I messed up my wrist a little. I would have my wrists constantly bent and tight in the same position to cart around those heavy appliances. It eventually started to hurt, and after realizing what my chiropractor did to me once to realign my knee, I decided to mimic him on my wrist. I just wrapped my hand around my wrist, gave a little tug, and I heard the crack sound. It became realigned and provided temporary relief. Then I began to flex the wrist in the opposite direction than what I had been flexing it. That corrected the muscle imbalance. Now it's all better.

The same problem was occurring when I started to develop carpel tunnel syndrome in my knuckles, from typing over a keyboard at a desk all day. I had my fingers constantly bent in the same position. I discovered that this position stretched out muscles that are responsible for pulling the fingers back (top of the forearm). So what did I do? I simply began flexing my fingers back as far as they would go, and did so for a few sets. If carpel tunnel ever rears its ugly head, I do this move on the fingers. No more carpel tunnel.

For your case, wherever the arthritis may be, you're going to want to find out the best way to counter the tension that the stronger muscles are putting on your joints. If you've had to hold a muscle in a fixed position for long periods of time, wouldn't it make sense to find a workout that will work against that muscle? Work the antagonistic muscle group. The balance will maintain proper alignment in the corresponding joint.

Here's the fun part. The spine is mainly affected by the hip. The hip has 18 muscles attached to it. Some of these muscles are very rarely used. Even when they are used, it's probably not for long or very rigorously. What's more fun, you are probably going to have to isolate each underdeveloped muscle in order to get it stronger. Compound moves tend to recruit muscles that are already overdeveloped, and continuing to strengthen them will not help the imbalance one bit. It will actually continue to hurt the joint. Isolation moves will call for some interesting workout positions. You will have several muscles to strengthen, which may take some funny positions.

Finding your Problem(s)

Chronic back, neck, joint, digestive, etc. discomfort and/or pain mostly boil down to the same problem – the imbalances around the hip bone. The muscle imbalances around the hip bone are causing bones elsewhere to shift. Again, as the hip goes, so goes the spine. The spine then tilts out of alignment; the leg bone can twist and stress out the knees. I've found that the hip and spine even affect the shoulder joint. If my hip becomes displaced, I'll usually feel looseness in the shoulder socket and pain where the joint meets the spine in the base of my neck.

What was happening, in my case, was the dominant side of my hip was being yanked down by the overdeveloped muscles surrounding it – the thigh, hip flexor/adductor/abductor, and back. My dominant leg was being pulled out of its socket. It appears to be a concerted effort, because when I work the weaker muscles that counter the stress, all these overdeveloped muscles start to stretch out at the same time. If feels really good when that happens. During the workout, I'll usually get involuntary spasms in certain muscles to restore the joints to their proper alignment. By the end of the workout, I'll feel like I have a totally new body. I'll start to feel some pleasing sensations in my nerves. It's quite soothing. Balancing and bending over becomes a little difficult, which is good. It's like a toddler learning to walk, and toddlers normally have perfect posture. It's all about posture.

This yanking down of the hip and leg separation can tilt the spine and cause all sorts of problems, including clicking, grinding, and pain in the neck; mid-back pain, low back pain, headaches and migraines, sinus interference; knee, ankle and shoulder pain; numbness, that tickling sensation in the inner ear; vision impairment, dry eye, receding hairline and baldness; enlarged (hyper stretched) prostate, and digestive and reproductive problems. These are all simply structural problems, caused by muscle imbalances in the core of your body.

Clicking, Grinding, and Pain in the Neck
If when you turn your head or breathe deeply you notice a clicking or grinding in the neck, you have a problem. The vertebrae are out of alignment. There *may* not be much or any pain, but letting it go will eventually cause some type of discomfort, maybe even arthritis in the neck. You must find out what you are doing to push these vertebrae, and/or the leg, out of alignment. The problem could even be a combination of factors, like it was for me.

Between the ages of about 18 and 21, my neck was in disturbing pain. It eventually brought me to tears one day on my drive home from college. I could not hold my neck up to drive, and that day it was unbearable. I attribute that debilitating condition to all the athletics and manual labor that stressed out and displaced my hip bone and spine, as well as all the sitting I had to do in college.

I eventually discovered that the bulk of the problem rested on the abdomen and dominant external oblique – the grinding seems to be caused by the oblique alone. The pelvis may play a smaller role as well. They seem to take the bulk of the stress from the overdeveloped legs and back, and be the cause of a lot of problems, as you'll soon see. When we sit, we typically lose posture and push the hip and spine out of alignment, weakening the core muscles attached to them. That's why I see a lot of people twist their neck as they sit. Our poor posture affects the upper spine. I also learned that simply walking wrongly can yank against muscles in the core. One real problem in the hip is, to some degree, that dislocation of the leg socket. Our overdeveloped leg muscles can really yank on that leg bone and pull on the socket. Add to that the toll sitting takes on that socket, and it sets us up real well for a slew of problems.

Muscle imbalances between the front and rear deltoids can also have an effect on the base of the neck, where the shoulder meets the spine. The position your arms are in as you work during the day could be hyper stretching an already underdeveloped rear deltoid. You could be holding up your arms for long periods of time, maybe holding them forward to type at a keyboard or something like that. This unnatural position and stretch of the read deltoid shifts the shoulder joint, which is connected to the upper spine.

Heavy weightlifting in the chest and shoulders may be pulling against weak rear deltoid, rotator cuff, and trapezius muscles. Strengthening the traps and weak rear deltoids will pull those shoulders right back where they belong, if this is your problem. Flexing the rotator cuffs in a backward motion may also benefit. I used to do countless chest exercises, which I finally found to be hurting my neck real bad. I found great relief when strengthening the under developed muscles in the core. There still existed some discomfort, so I combined those core exercises with rear deltoid and trap muscle strengthening, and sealed the comfort.

A muscle imbalance between the biceps and triceps can be yet another problem. I used to do a ton of biceps curls and not as much inner triceps extensions to match the strength. So my shoulders would be pulled forward even harder.

I will show you how to correct these kinds of problems and guide you to make sure they never resurface.

The other reasons for bad neck pain would be the result of a fall or car accident/whiplash, probably set up by hip displacement. Some kind of sudden jerk of the neck can force the vertebrae out of alignment. To decrease the potential for accident-caused misalignments, or slash the time it will take to recover from one, I will show you later in the guide how to get hip and spinal stability from core workouts.

Hip displacement is likely the precursor to neck and back pain from accidents. Some times you may not even know you've had a hip or spine problem, until you actually have an accident. Growing up I didn't have chronic pain, but I did have some discomfort and I noticed some functions around the hip were interfered with. It may take an accident to push the hip and spine over the edge. Quite often, chiropractor visits alone do not reverse the stress that's been building up over the years in your hip and spine. If you're still in pain or discomfort after a couple months seeing a chiropractor, you have a muscle imbalance or two, or several, to correct.

Pain in the Middle Back
I once heard of someone who, no matter how many times they would go to their chiropractor, would always have to have the middle back section of their spine adjusted. It was constantly out of alignment (This sort of gets me wondering about chiropractors. Mine never could inform me of exactly why my bones kept falling out of alignment. He would just keep adjusting the alignments, visit after visit). This can be quite a painful condition. I know from experience.

This chronic condition is caused by - take a guess - a muscle imbalance around the hip. Posture is wrecked because of it, allowing vertebrae to slide out of alignment and pinch the nerves. The 6-pack abdomen seems to be the major player in mid back pain, whether you're ambidextrous or not. My father is ambidextrous, and he never had any structural problems until his 60s. But when it finally did happen, it was brutal. He said it felt like someone stabbing him in the middle of his back, at the bottom of his shoulder blade. I've concluded that since weight is evenly distributed on both sides of his (ambidextrous) body, the problem must be up the middle - the abdomen.

Low Back Pain
The most common of all pain man suffers from. If you sit in an office all day, or sit anywhere all day, and you have not the knowledge of the natural curves of the spine and how to keep them aligned, you're putting a lot of pressure on your hip and spine. Like I mentioned in the "let my body go" web site, sitting for long periods of time is <u>brutal</u> on the hip and spine. When you sit, you typically stretch just about all the underdeveloped muscles around the hip, and straighten the curve in your spine. This puts way more stress on the lower spine than standing (which is why I now look for opportunities to do some of my office work standing).

Unless all the muscles in your core are tight and balanced, the vertebrae are aligned, and you have the correct posture, you've got a problem. This is why the number of office workers with back pain is so high. They're in the prime positions to force their vertebrae and hip out of alignment and pinch the nerves. They just don't know it. "A total of 56% of BCA chiropractors highlighted that those who work in an office were more vulnerable to becoming victims of back pain".[1] "Approximately 31 million visits were made to physicians' offices due to back problems in 2003, including more than 10 million visits for low back problems."[2] Most, if not all, are avoidable.

One of my sisters told us once about her back pain. She mentioned a hump on the right side of her lower back. That was her overdeveloped, dominant back muscle. The right side was naturally bearing the bulk of her upper body load her whole life, and when she bent over to do her job. This causes stress to the hip and spine, and it's probably the most common overdeveloped muscle in the body. My back was the same way. Until I knew better, my body was heavily dominated by the right side. Ambidextrous people probably don't suffer too much from muscle imbalances like this. Two people in my family are ambidextrous, and until my Dad was in his 60's, neither exhibited any kind of structural problem.

Here, you'll be shown what you need to know - how to support your spine by strengthening your core, and how to sit, walk and sleep in order to maintain your proper spinal alignment. With a strong core and proper posture, you can get away with sitting and bending in any position you want (but too much of that in one day will eventually work against the strength you've built up). What I've just told you and what I will tell you below are things I don't think chiropractors even know about.

If you work out a lot and work your abs regularly, you may have a problem. You've probably been working your abs wrong. I've read about guys who work out yet have back pain when they do their ab routine. This is because 1) their vertebrae are forced out of their natural curvature by the crunching motion, and 2) they are involuntarily jacking up their hip flexors and adductors doing traditional crunches on traditional ab benches.

By doing so many crunches and the likes, you are actually working to straighten out that curve in your spine (forcing the vertebrae further and further out of alignment), stressing out the hip and spine and putting more and more pressure on the nerves down there. The hip flexors are already strong muscles. We use them every day to walk and run. Traditional crunches just further strengthen them. The pressure is always going to be there outside of the gym because, as we all know, muscles get, and stay, more tense as they are used more and more. This keeps constant pressure on the nerves that run out through those vertebrae in the spine, resulting in the pain. Ab workouts can fix poor posture, but only if they're done properly. Coming up, I'll show you how to do them properly.

In general, as I have probably made evident, doing a lot of front body workouts, without doing a similar amount of antagonistic workouts, will really yank on the natural curves of your spine. And if it's not clear yet, most imbalances are between the legs, back and core muscles. Focusing on frontal workouts in the chest, front deltoids, thighs and hip flexors will force your upper body into sort of a hunched position. Sitting in the office all day with your hip and shoulders tucked forward has the same effect. Doing manual, back busting labor has a negative effect as well. The spine does not agree with these activities at all – man's price for the privilege of being the upright species.

Unless and until you start to strengthen the most neglected muscles in your body around the spine and hip, you will always be putting pressure on the vertebrae, and they will constantly be forced to slip, and stay, out of alignment. I see a lot of people walking around with their hip sort of tucked forward, and some with shoulders that are slouched forward. I always wonder how much pain they're in. Doing more work on the neglected muscles than you do on your overdeveloped back and legs will keep the pressure off your spine. I will show you exactly what to do to work these neglected muscles.

It is likely a combination of weak muscle groups contributing to your poor posture and low back pain, starting with the dominant external oblique, with lesser help from the pelvis and abdomen (6 pack). Six months or so into my chiropractor routine, I tried out an ab exercise I had never tried before and thought would help my back pain. I tried what they call the Russian plate twist. It's where you sit on an ab bench holding a weight plate in front of you, and rotate that plate around your body, from 9 o'clock to 3 o'clock. Immediately upon doing this exercise, the lower half of my spine cracked. That began my relief from low back pain. Judging from this, the dominant external oblique appears to be a major contributor. This Russian plate twist flexes the obliques well. I don't recommend this exercise as it typically incorporates the hip flexors and puts your body into the crunched position. It also flexes the non dominant external oblique if you twist in both directions. But if you're desperate for a quick fix to the low back pain, go for it. Just keep your hip flexors relaxed. Your pelvis will make up for it. And flex only your dominant side. Put the plate over on the non dominant side. I'll show you the best way to isolate the dominant external oblique in the exercise section.

Doing more work on the neglected muscles than you do on your overdeveloped back and legs will keep the pressure off your spine. Together, they'll slide the back of your hip up into your lower back, and suck your mid section into the hip socket better, restoring the lower curve of your spine. I will show you exactly what to do to work the neglected muscles.

Hip Pain
Hip displacement is really the cause of almost all these other structural problems, but it's usually not painful. If it's painful, you're probably feeling it in the area at the top of your butt. My hip displacement never became painful until the tail end of my recovery. I was just flexing on my ab chair one day when I felt a sharp pain at the top of my bum. It felt like someone was jabbing a screwdriver into my socket. And it was on the non dominant side.

In my experience, exercising the abdomen dominant external oblique seemed to be the solution to the painful part of hip displacement. I thought it strange that pain on my non-dominant side was being caused by hyper-stretched muscles on the dominant side. The abdomen and pelvis probably contribute to some degree as well.

Shoulder Problems

Athletes and office workers tend to put so much stress on their shoulder that it becomes loose, weak, or very painful. One problem is a constant stretching of the rear deltoid, rotator cuff, and trapezius muscles. Heavy weightlifting, constant throwing, and sitting at a desk all day with your arms forward can all stress out the rear deltoid and rotator cuff.

Amazingly, poor posture in the spine, aided by hip displacement, can affect the shoulder socket as well. I see the shoulder/neck complaint often from fellow coworkers, and some times myself, who are forced to sit at a desk all day to do our jobs. Improve posture – core muscles – and you'll improve how the shoulders set in their sockets. This condition seems to start with the pelvis.

Headaches, Sciatica, Sinus Pressures, that Tickling Sensation in the Inner Ear, Chronic Dry Eye, and Hair Loss.

If you suffer from any of these, your nerve supply is being pinched. As I told you earlier, your nerves run through all the vertebrae in your spine, top to bottom. If the vertebrae are out of alignment, they are pinching these nerves. Bad things can happen when nerves are pinched.

A former coworker has a son who has chronic migraine headaches. I pretty much knew what the problem was, but I asked her anyway if her son works out a lot. He does. He was a runt trying to get huge, like me. He was doing a lot of crunches and the typical guy workouts. It got so bad he had to go see specialists in other states to see if they could help (this after I had already explained to her exactly what the problem was). All they could tell her was – 'his spine is messed up, and the nerve is being pinched'. No kidding. What's causing that to happen? Bad posture and spine misalignment from all his improper exercises. To this day, three years later, I don't believe he's fixed his problem.

I had a brief stint with migraines. One day my chiropractor went to adjust the very top of my spine and noticed something. He asked me if I had been having headaches recently. I answered in the affirmative and he adjusted me. The headaches left and that was one of my last adjustments in his office. It was around this point that I finally began to reverse the muscle imbalances around my hip and spine. Headaches come few and far between now.

If by some chance the top of your spine is out of alignment and needs manipulation to stop the headaches, you can try one trick yourself. It's a simple twist of the head and top of the neck. You can put your chin in your hand and twist your head toward your dominant side until you hear a crack. You might see people do it on occasion. I came across my brother's friend one day who was having a migraine attack. I showed him this technique and he was grossed out when he heard the crack. When I turned around to walk away, I heard a crack from him. He got relief. One night my 6-year old nephew was having neck pain. I had him twist his head a little like this and his neck cracked. No more neck pain.

I lived with chronic sinus problems for years as a teenager. Every time the seasons changed, I would get a sinus infection. But a few prayers and a phone call later, that period of time was put to an end. I found the right chiropractor. As soon as I started in on his program, relief came and the sinus infections never returned. Other painful conditions were still there, but not as bad as before. I still had work to do to reverse the stress I had put on my spine and joints over the years.

Headache and sinus problems seem to stem from a weakened dominant external oblique, with maybe smaller contributions from the pelvis (I feel like a broken record). If you are suffering from these conditions, you can do the techniques I will show you to strengthen these muscles.

It wasn't until I started properly flexing these muscles that my sciatica started to go away for good. Another trick that should help a bunch if you suffer with sciatica is to jam your dominant leg back and up into its socket. Especially if I'm sitting, if I feel the sciatic nerve start to lose itself or become uncomfortable, I'll just jam that leg back and up into its socket real good. That move slides the back of the hip into the lower back and improves posture. The pelvis seems to be the weakened muscle that needs strengthening in this case. Strengthen your pelvis – in the weird way I'll detail in the exercise section – and that should end at least the bulk of your sciatica. The dominant external oblique may play a smaller role in sciatic nerve interference, just not nearly as much as the pelvis.

The pelvis seems to play a big role in the inner ear, tickling sensation issue.

It's tough to pin point chronic dry eye. It seems to a combination dominant external oblique and abdomen problem. I suffered with chronic dry eye for a couple years. It began when I started sitting in a chair all day earning a living, and it got so bad I started to develop sties in my eyelids. Some got so large they had to be surgically removed.

Again, a receding hair line (balding) seems to be caused by a weakened abdomen.

Restless Leg Syndrome
Another chronic structural problem I've suffered with, on and off. Your legs feel like they have to move or kick when you're just lying there. It's nerve interference, of course. It's the position our bed and bum pushes our hip into when we lay down that's putting stress on the nerves. This position is brutal on the hip. The jury is still out on this one. It seems to be brought on by a weakened dominant oblique. But it could be a combination of muscles. I'm just not positive yet.

The sensation runs down the overdeveloped hip flexors, and the core muscles pull against the flexors. It's pretty much the dominant leg bone being sucked out of the hip socket. We use our flexors all day every day, since we learned to walk. That's a lot of strengthening in that area. We rarely use the muscles that counter them. If you're heavily dominated by one side of your body for walking or other moves, you work that hip flexor way too hard. It's causing an unnatural position, yanking that leg out of its socket.

If I'm lying in bed and I feel RLS coming on, I'll typically flex the abdomen, pelvis and/or external oblique. Some times I'll have to get up to flex and reset the hip. My hip shifts, posture improves, and the sensation goes away.

Indigestion, Constipation/Irregularity, Acid Reflux, Ulcers, Enlarged Prostate
Initially, I wasn't going to insert this section if I ever wrote this book. "Too embarrassing," I thought. Then, I heard on the evening news one day a guy call 911. "My wife hasn't gone to the bathroom in like a month", I heard. I thought, "man, someone has to shine some light in this darkness". Some estimates say that over 4 million people in the US use laxatives frequently.

Running along your hip and spine is your digestive system. This long tube is attached to the bones it runs along, and the reproductive muscles are attached to the end of it. So, you have this matrix of digestive, skeletal, muscular, reproductive and nervous systems, all coming together in the hip. When the hip and spine fall out of their alignment, the bones put pressure on all these systems. When it's bad enough, the digestive and reproductive systems will be interfered with to the point they may partially block the food from exiting. Amazingly, this stress also appears to affect the whole system - causing indigestion, acid reflux, and, from what I've experienced, ulcers. This is the cause of an enlarged (hyper stretched) prostate as well.

Again, sitting is brutal on the hip and spine. Sitting takes that big curve in the back and tries to straighten it. Sitting on the "John" is no exception.

All you need to do is strengthen the weak supporting muscles in your core to push the hip bone and spine back into their natural alignment, and you take the stress back off the digestive and reproductive systems. That's it – improve your posture. Get that big curve back. Suck your legs up into their sockets. The tubes will open back up and digestion will flow perfectly. Just follow the upcoming techniques I outline. Strengthen those neglected, weak core muscles. This will push the hip bone back against the overdeveloped muscles in your legs and back, restoring the natural curvature of your spine.

The problem seems to be a combination of the weaker, underdeveloped muscles surrounding the hip and spine. I call them the big 3 – the dominant external oblique, pelvis and abdomen. These muscles took some serious abuse in my body. If you're ambidextrous and you have digestive problems, it's probably just your pelvis and abdomen. I know for a fact a weak abdomen causes indigestion.

You may have to flex some of these underdeveloped muscles even when you're sitting, on the John or anywhere, to improve posture while you're sitting.

Doctors say that two bowel movements in a day is natural and ideal. Growing up I wouldn't have believed that. I wouldn't go more than once a day, some times every other day. But once I began to strengthen some underdeveloped muscles that are attached to the digestive pipes, I started going twice a day, like a baby, just like they say. One of the few times the doctors get it right. 18

Opening up the digestive channels like this will also allow for better digestion and circulation. I found my mental performance, focus, blood flow, and overall energy levels to improve drastically when I began to focus on the neglected, weak muscles in my core. No more indigestion, reflux, gas, or even bloating.

You may have heard or seen programs that tell us how our colon can build up with old food and toxins. Again, this problem is caused by interference from the surrounding misaligned bones. When you strengthen the neglected muscles in your core and smooth out the digestive tract, you'll probably soon have a pretty large bowel movement as this old waste is finally flushed.

You may have noticed that the pelvis, abdomen, and oblique are the common factors in hip and spine structural problems (for people who aren't ambidextrous). They also happen to be the first to fail and stretch back out in supporting the hip and spine during usual, every day activity. I can take a casual walk the wrong way and they will become stretched out via their antagonistic muscle groups in the back and legs. If this recovery process were a house, these areas would be the foundation. You're going to want to start with them in the upcoming sections of recovery exercises. It is going to take serious work to strengthen them.

Tennis Elbow
Fortunately, my stint with this problem was brief. It stings a lot. I found the solution by accident. It's actually a rotation of the forearm that's stressing out the elbow. That's apparently why they call it tennis elbow. Tennis players constantly have their forearm rotated out to hold the racket in the right position for play.

To fix, just rotate your forearm in the opposite direction you would have it if you were holding a tennis racket to swing it. Maybe add a dumbbell and rest your forearm on a bench for more resistance. At some point during or after the exercise your elbow should crack. Do a few sets every day until the pain doesn't appear any more.

Bum Knees
After visiting my chiropractor 3 times a week for a couple months, I learned how to mimic his moves on my own bones. Some how I discovered I could twist my knees in a certain

motion and crack them (I used to have a loose knee). Later, I learned to crack my ankles in the same motion, usually at the same time as my knee. All I do is plant the bad leg and rotate the rest of my body back and away from it, taking some pressure off of that leg at the same time. Try it, and you should crack it. You can probably crack it every day, thanks to all the stress we continually put on our hip.

My step dad injured his knee really bad at work one day. While visiting with the family, I showed this technique to him. He tried it and, lo and behold, the knee cracked and it's never hurt him since (that I know of).

It appears there could be two reasons for knee problems. My step dad's case was an accident. It wasn't a slow approach to knee pain. The other reason would be a slower breakdown of knee support, from hip stress. It could even be a combination of both. If it's hip stress in your case, you're going to need to strengthen the weak muscles around the hip. It will restore your knees and keep them strong for life. The abdomen is probably the primary contributor to such a shift in the hip area putting stress on the knees. The external oblique could be contributing as well. Another small factor could be the dominant hamstring. The hamstring is responsible for curling the leg. If you have super strong thighs, this could be a problem for you.

The hamstrings seem to have a special benefit to the knees. They pull against the flexors, adductors and IT band. Whenever I isolate them with leg curls (which is rare), it feels like I put a set of Dr. Scholl's gel inserts in my knees. They feel fine without working the hamstrings, but when I do they feel even better. When I'm lying in bed, it's actually a pleasing sensation. You'll see how to strengthen them later.

Pain in the Toes
At times my toes used to get kind of irritated. Being one of the last chronic pain conditions I suffered from, I knew quickly what the problem was. I figured all I had to do was adjust their

alignments and flex them in the opposite direction than what I had been doing my whole life (grinding them down into the ground for balance and grip). Once again, it was a muscle imbalance. I told you I suffered with just about every pain you can think of.

To adjust the toes, I usually just take the other foot, step on them a little with the heel, and pull to straighten them out. I'll hear a crack or two, and then I work them in the opposite direction for a while. Relief without the pills, creams, drinks, or ointments. That pinky toe is kind of difficult to work, though.

Carpel Tunnel Syndrome

Your knuckles feel like they have sandpaper in them. Mine sure did. Although I didn't suffer with this problem nearly as long as I've suffered with most structural problems, I still suffered. How often do you straighten your fingers back or bend them back, in the opposite direction you hold things or keep them over a keyboard? Never, huh? Well, that's the problem. It's a muscle imbalance. The muscles in the front of your fingers, hands and arms are tight. The muscles behind are hyper stretched.

You may not have carpel tunnel, but just a chronically sore knuckle – maybe the middle? This happens to me on occasion. I know two people who've had this problem, and I showed each exactly what to do to stop it. Neither even bothered to move their fingers in the direction I was telling them, as far as I know (some times I wonder if people initially don't do what I tell them, but then they think about it later, it sinks in, and they try it). Within the first 5 minutes of me flexing my fingers back several times as far as they would go, relief came. That's all you need to do, strengthen the back of your hands and forearms, and straighten out the fingers.

You may have seen someone on TV or in a movie - right before they're about to start in on some work - lock their fingers, put their palms forward and stretch the fronts of their fingers, hands and forearms that way. That's a great way to work against carpel tunnel.

Numbness, Loss of Feeling, Pinched Nerve

These three are basically the same. A pinched nerve is a longer lasting effect, and can be painful, though. These are all caused by pressure on the nerve. That pressure is coming from bones that are pushed out of their natural alignment. In one of my more unpleasant cases, I would wake up with a pinched nerve along my forearm, hand and finger. It wasn't very painful, but more of a dull throb. It did get in the way if I needed to use that hand and finger a lot. In my sleep, I would subconsciously bend my arms and place my hands on my chest. I still catch myself doing it on occasion.

Whatever nerve is painful or numb in your case, you must determine what position you are holding or placing your bones or joints that is causing this numbness or pinched nerve. You could be doing it in your sleep. You could be doing it while working or playing.

What do I Need to do to Get Rid of the Problems (Fix my Vertebrae)?

It's time to push back. I will show you how you can catapult the core recovery process by strengthening the correct muscles attached to your hip and spine.

Techniques to Lasting Pain Relief

The remaining part of this e-book is like pure gold. I'm going to give you the greatest tips, tricks, and techniques for lasting comfort that you can get. There's nothing like it anywhere. No matter what your occupation, I give you the steps you can take to rid and keep yourself from pain and discomfort, slash chiropractor visits, and save yourself boo coos of dollars.

Implement the Correct Postures

Take this piece of advice with you wherever you are - do not hunch to the best of your ability. Remember, your spine has curves to it, and your hip needs to slide back to accommodate the lower curve. Your spine is kept best aligned when these curves are allowed to be curvy. When we are seated, if we're not careful, we can lose as much as 30% of our curve. You need to minimize the pressure put on it. This may not be easy at first, but after you do some of the upcoming workouts in the next section, it will be natural and easy. Your hip will slide back up into your lower back, your back will arch, and your chest will stick out.

A rule of thumb I go by, to maintain perfect alignment, is to make a habit of *emphasizing* the lower curve in my spine. The best way to accomplish this, when you're walking, is to allow your buttocks to sort of stick out. Don't kick so hard to walk, but make shorter steps. Your feet may kind of shuffle walking like this, but it's worth it for the relief. If you can feel a very slight stretch in back muscles, hip flexors, adductors and thighs, when you're sitting or standing, you're doing it perfectly. This slight stretch is actually critical. It helps the very lowest vertebrae in the curve to stay locked in alignment. Remember, an overdeveloped, tight back is dangerous to the spine.

I actually had to learn how to walk, how to sit, and how to sleep properly. I guess there really is an art form to everything.

A poor posture will give you problems in the curves of the spine. Without implementing the correct posture, the hip bone and vertebrae will always fall out of alignment. If you constantly sit with your upper body bent forward, or hunched, you'll put a bunch of stress on the curves and hip.

I stick my chin up to emphasize the curve in my neck. This helps maintain open channels for the nerves which control vision and tear production. I will also sort of tilt my head back a little, and maybe squeeze the back of my neck. You may hear a little crunching back there if you do that. That's just the vertebrae being put back into the proper alignment. This tilt improved my vision a little. I also noticed one day that this squeeze of the neck muscles stopped an annoying ringing in my head I woke up to.

If you're a weightlifter who tenses the front of his neck while lifting, I recommend squeezing the back of your neck while lifting from now on, instead of the front. It will neutralize and reverse some tension you may be putting on your upper spine.

Sitting Posture
It's just about impossible to sit while keeping the curvature in your lower back maintained. This position accommodates your hip flexors and adductors, shortening them. They need to be stretched back out.

When you sit, I recommend first relaxing your entire body. Lean against the back rest, flex all the underdeveloped muscles - the pelvis, abdomen, and dominant external oblique - to push your hip and spine into the proper alignment, and then sit up. That should get your posture perfect for sitting. Your shoulders should be pushed back, the back of your hip wanting to slide up into your lower back, and your spine wanting to be curved. That technique can really make a difference, and you can do it whenever you want.

To reduce the impact as much as possible, your legs are going to want to be pushed back and up into the sockets as good as possible, especially your dominant leg. When your upper legs feel like they want to kick back against the chair and into their sockets, you then should feel the back of your hip want to slide up into your lower back. Let it. Your upper body should then straighten up like a board, and the curve in your lower back should be restored at least a little. This position helps the hamstrings, too.

I find sitting closer to the edge of a chair some times is best to accommodate this position of the hip and spine. It's nigh impossible to keep the leg bones up into their sockets properly while sitting all the way back in a seat. My upper body wants to lean back to accommodate the leg socket, but if my hip is closer to the edge of the seat, the legs can be lower and sucked into the sockets better. It may not be good to have a fat wallet in your rear pocket while you're sitting. I found out it can help wreck the hip.

Sleep Posture
Just as important as the sitting posture is that which you use while you sleep. For eight or so hours, your spine is pretty much in the same position. If it's in the wrong position, you can kiss comfort for the upcoming day good-bye, unless you can maintain perfect posture during the day to compensate. If in the right position, you'll wake up every time feeling like a million bucks. During the process of restoring the spine, with the right sleeping posture, you'll feel better and better each successive morning you wake up.

I recommend you keep from lying on your side when you sleep. To maximize spinal comfort, make sure the lower curve is maintained, at least a little. Don't sleep in the fetal position. It accommodates the hip adductors, and pulls on your lower curve.

When you lie down in bed maybe flex all your weaker core muscles. The back of your hip should slide up a little, your butt should press down into the mattress and your spine should curve back. That way the spine and joints stay in their alignment all night. This will probably allow you to sleep better as well. If you suffer from RLS, this will keep it from creeping up on you in bed.

If you really want to treat yourself nice, there's even a way to accommodate the hip even better, when you sleep on your back. Your legs are not meant to be dead straight. There's a natural, slight bend in the knees and you might want to help that happen while you sleep. Just stick something under them so they're slightly bent - maybe a small pillow or towel. You can use whatever feels good.

If you like to lie on your stomach while sleeping, this is no good. This will set you up for major pressure on the hip and spine. You must lie on the back.

At first these new positions may be uncomfortable for you, just because they're different. They were for me. But I knew I had to get them down or else I would never make it to optimal spinal strength and pain free living. Force yourself to make the transition, and before you know it you'll be sleeping through the night like a rock, and waking up every morning feeling like a million bucks. The only downside is you'll be so relaxed you won't want to get up out of bed. Make adjustments until you're perfectly comfortable lying on your back. You may need to flex some of those underdeveloped muscles to fix your posture and slide your butt back while you're lying there. Do whatever it takes. Getting a night of quality sleep will prepare you well for the challenging day ahead.

Remember, pay attention to detail. I like to do everything to allow for the spinal curves - sit, sleep, and walk. It repels injury and pain, keeps me at peak performance levels for every day tasks, and helps digestion, which allows for perfect energy flow in the mind. If there is anything you're subtly doing in your postures that pushes, and keeps, your hip and vertebrae out of alignment, change the position.

I will discuss walking posture after the workout section.

Balancing out Muscle Imbalances
If you love to lift weights, you're probably a victim of muscle imbalances. For example, if you like to jack up your chest and deltoids to look buff and impress the ladies (like I used to), you could be developing some bad muscle imbalances around the neck. When I learned this was what was causing some of my neck and shoulder pain, I had to totally change my workout. My front deltoids and chest were too strong for my upper back and shoulder muscles.

One of the imbalances I had developed - and this is probably really common for anyone, let alone weightlifters - was between my chest, front and lateral deltoids, and my traps and rear deltoids.

Another common imbalance I've noticed occurs among squat lifters. I used to do squats myself. I read one story how a person was doing squats one day and had something shift in her hip. Jacking up the thighs will put serious pressure on the core muscles. I don't work my legs, or back, for nothing any more. They've had, and continue to get, all the exercise they'll need for a lifetime.

If you have developed a muscle imbalance and are putting unruly stress on joints or vertebrae, you're now going to have to work to stretch the overdeveloped muscles, and build up the hyper stretched, weaker antagonistic muscle group(s) to match the dominance and keep stress off your vertebrae and joints. Here, I'll show you some techniques which can neutralize muscle imbalances.

Also, if you have spotted which muscle groups are too strong for their counterparts, you may be able to just sit there and tense them up any time you want. This technique works well for me, as a temporary relief, until I can do a full workout.

To do these workouts at home, you will need an Ab Chair or Ab Lounge mechanism, dumbbells and maybe a bench and ankle weights. Altogether, if you get a 40 lb set of adjustable dumbbells, 5-10 lb ankle weights, a bench, and an ab chair mechanism, it shouldn't cost much more than a couple hundred bucks. And this combo (as long as you're creative) can take the place of many super expensive sets of home gyms and equipment. If you're a member of a gym, you can use machines instead of dumbbells, or both, and anything else it has to do all the following moves. You may have ideas of better moves to do for any muscle groups. Go for it. Improvise... guess, test, and revise... be creative!

If you're going to just stick with the bare minimum investment, make sure it's the ab chair/lounge mechanism. That is essential. Some people have a hard time bringing themselves to even spend that much. But, it's either pay a chunk now, or keep paying many, many smaller chunks the rest of your life. $80 turns out to be a fraction of the cost for the latter. It will seriously be one of the best investments of your life, if not the best.

Keep in mind that strengthening one neglected muscle group in your core may slightly and inadvertently work against another weaker muscle group that you intend to strengthen. It's like taking two steps forward and one step back. To neutralize this effect, you may want to exercise all the muscles in your core on the same day. That will probably keep you from taking a step back.

Core Workouts for Spine and Joint Support

The ab chair mechanism (aka ab lounge) is critical here. It will turbo-charge your campaign to stop and reverse hip and spine misalignment. The ab chair saved my life.

As moves get easier, you will need to add weight for more resistance. I usually strap on some ankle weights and hold a dumbbell or two against the top of the chair as I'm flexing.

Stay away from traditional core exercises that personal trainers like to make us do. Traditional workouts for core strength do not isolate the core muscles, and sometimes involve crunching motions. They're almost all compound moves. They will utilize already overdeveloped muscles, like the thighs and hip abductors, and continue the pain and discomfort being put on the nervous, digestive and reproductive systems. You do not want to do body balancing moves, or run, ever again. These moves will cause more harm than good, even if you're working core muscles at the same time.

I experience relief when I strengthen the 6-pack abs, pelvis and dominant external oblique. They appear to make up for most of the slack. When working these, I can actually feel the hip bone push against my thighs, hip adductors, abductors, and flexors; and back muscles. These over developed muscles begin to stretch back out.

All of the following workouts together may not be possible for you to do, for a lack of equipment or whatever, but do what you can. A friend of mine flexes these muscles lying on his back on the floor. That was his exercise. That did help him get relief. Trust me, even one of these exercises can yield dividends in back pain and joint pain relief.

It will take serious focus to isolate and control these muscles because of the stretched positions they've been under for so long. Try not to get lazy while working them. I recommend at least 3 or 4 sets for whatever muscle group you work. The more the merrier. Like anything, the more you invest, the greater your dividends.

6 Pack Abs and Pelvis

Ironically, it takes front side strength to make the back side feel better. When you flex your abs and pelvis to reverse this stress on the hip and back, you should feel all the overdeveloped muscles in your legs and back really stretch out, all at the same time. If you find yourself needing to add weight to the top of the chair for more resistance, you will probably need to put on a set of 5-10 pound ankle weights to balance the chair. Also, counting each rep helps maintain focus so we get the most out of these workouts. I notice if I let my mind wander, I slack.

Isolating each of these muscles seems to be the effective way to work them and push that hip bone against the overdeveloped muscles. It really pushes the bone against muscles on the dominant side. Flexing the core muscles will actually slide the back of your hip up into your lower back and force a better posture.

Sit on the chair, ankles resting on the foot rest. You're not going to flex the same way as you would doing traditional crunches. Your upper body isn't going to come forward very much at all. You are just going to <u>put the muscle on stretch</u>, then <u>press your six pack flat against your spine</u>, driving the seat of the chair down - pulling against the over developed legs and back muscles, and sliding the back of your hip bone up into your lower back. It's going to force your butt back and curve the lower spine <u>while you flex</u>. You should feel your hip slide to your dominant side a little and some overdeveloped muscle groups stretch out real good. It will slightly move in the same motion you'd make if you were working your external oblique. It pulls the dominant side of your hip and leg bone up into the socket better. It will also jam the back of your hip bone into your lower back real good and force a nice posture. You should feel the small of your back, right behind the back of your hip bone, stretch out. But you must absolutely do these moves so that a big curve in your lower spine ensues. If you don't feel that big curve develop, you're doing it wrong. Remember, don't crunch – just squeeze the individual muscle and push it toward your spine. Posture will ensue.

Focusing on the pelvis, just drive your bum and the seat of the chair straight down. It's going to be like a short jackknife kind of move. You should start to feel the back of your hip bone drive up into your lower back, forming a nice arch, and your legs want to be pushed back and into their sockets better. If you're not ambidextrous, your mid section should start to get crooked while your hip bone is driven back against the dominant muscles yanking on it. Really concentrate on sliding the back of your hip bone into the very lower part of your back, sucking your legs into their sockets better, and allowing those inner adductor muscles to be stretched out. It may take some practice to perfect this move. It took me years. And, for me at least, this is typically the first muscle to slack during every day sitting, bending, lifting, walking, etc.

On the abdomen, use the deep inside of that six pack to pull against those inner adductors and the lower back, and pull your legs into their sockets real good. It's going to slide your bum up toward your lower back, not crunch forward. Now, if you have a dominant side to your body, you will actually have to go so far as to flex extra hard the half of your 6 pack which is on that dominant side. This is done at the tail end of the abdomen flex. So, right as you're coming to the full flex of the abdomen, focus on continuing to flex the half of your 6 pack on your dominant side. That is a very important little move. This all may take some time and practice to master, but once you master it, it feels so much better. When the back of your hip drives up into your lower back muscles and wants to slide toward your dominant side, you're there. When your leg bones get sucked up into their sockets better, you're there. That's the feeling you'll always want to have from now on.

You may also be able to get away with flexing both the pelvis and abdomen to work them. I don't think it's as effective, after testing these moves for years, but it seems to provide a little benefit if done properly. Just flex them so that the back of your hip slides up your lower back – no crunching.

Again, the ab chair is the only way to flex the pelvis and abdomen while maintaining perfect posture at the same time. It's basically the only way to reconstruct the underdeveloped muscles to permanently restore posture.

You will want to make these moves on your pelvis and abs in just about any position your body is in from now on – from sleeping to standing. It may take some practice to perfect these moves. Play around with them. Focus on the muscle you're working on.

Doing sit-ups on the floor or ab bench still has a benefit or two, provided you don't utilize your hip flexors/adductors at all. It provides much more resistance than you'll receive from the ab chair. It's still awkward for the spine, forcing the upper half forward into that unnatural position. Just keep your back relatively straight, and don't go all the way forward. One way I accomplished this move – when I used to do traditional crunches - is to simply stick my legs under a bed. That keeps them stuck so I don't have to use my flexors/adductors. The benefit in this move is the resistance, as well as the stretching that results in the hip flexors/adductors. You'll definitely have to work your dominant external oblique after you do traditional sit ups. The crunching motion works against it.

Be careful using the foot rest on the ab chair. It's a fantastic mechanism, but it's not fool proof. Doing certain moves will mildly stretch out other underdeveloped muscles. Be sure to rest your ankles on the foot rest, and not put your feet on it like the models in the ads do.

Your mid section may become naturally inclined to push itself into a slightly crooked position (in addition to sliding the back of your hip bone up) while doing core workouts. It'll be stretching out your back and non-dominant external oblique. That's a good thing, especially if you suffer from headaches. It's the way for your body to push the hip bone back against the overdeveloped muscles and provide relief for your hyper stretched core. It shortens the dominant side, while stretching everything else. You should get an involuntary muscle spasm in an attempt to suck the dominant side of your hip and leg bone up into the socket.

If you're ambidextrous, you probably won't have to worry about this weird crooked position. Also, you probably won't have to go any further than these exercises to find relief from your chronic structural problem.

Dominant Side External Oblique
The external obliques are the groups of muscles on the sides of your core, between the hip and ribs. Here's where it gets interesting. Unless you're ambidextrous, you don't want to do both external obliques. You only need to work the dominant side. Here's why:

Remember how I told you the overdeveloped muscles on my dominant side – like the back, thigh, abductor, flexor and adductor – used to yank that side of my hip down? That yank stretches out the dominant side oblique. As a result, it shortens the non dominant oblique, accommodating it well, so that it will never have to be strengthened (you need it stretched back out). The hip bone is tilting, stretching one oblique while accommodating the other. The pelvis, abs, and external oblique all aid in pushing the hip back up and relieving the dominant oblique. You really need to strengthen all to keep the hip up into its socket properly. This will keep the spine from tilting as well. It will push against the back, thighs, hip flexors, abductors, and adductors. Remember, as the hip goes, so goes the spine. It really takes a concerted effort from all the underdeveloped muscles to reverse the stress.

This muscle can be tricky. It took my years to perfect the move. To work the dominant side oblique, sit on the ab chair, tilted over between 45 and 90 degrees to the back rest, with the dominant side of your body up and off the seat. Put this oblique on stretch, and drive the seat of the chair down, squeezing the whole oblique, top to bottom - bringing that side of your hip up into its socket. Push the seat of the chair straight down to the ground and flex directly against the back and leg muscles. Flex so that your leg bone is sucked up into its socket better. I call this flex 'n lock. If you do it right, you should soon get an involuntary muscle spasm working against just about all of the overdeveloped muscles – low back, hip flexors, adductors, abductors, and thighs. It should feel like you're stretching the back muscles along your lower spine (that's a good thing).

You should feel this new position of your hip bone pull against the very inner adductor muscles, some times referred to as the groin. You should also feel your butt stick back real far, and your spine get that big curve in it. The back of your hip is sliding up the lower back. This should all feel really good.

When you get up off the chair, you should feel your upper body pull back. Notice how big the arch in your lower back becomes. When you go to walk, it will feel like trying to walk like a baby. If you've had hip problems, you may have experienced your dominant hip dragging behind the other side when you walk. Flexing this oblique and the pelvis and abdomen will suck that dominant hip up and into its socket.

I made a video demonstrating these main exercises for hip alignment:
https://www.youtube.com/watch?v=v2bRn4c7Kks

If you still feel any awkwardness in the knees or hip after doing all these exercises, then leg curls may be the last piece of the puzzle. If you run a lot or lift heavy weights for squat lifting, this could be a problem for you. All those extensions in the thighs with little to no flexing in the opposite direction will certainly stress out your hip and knees. Find a leg curl machine and do the basic lifts, with good posture.

When doing these core workouts, you may feel your shoulders set differently, with your chest stretching out. This is good. This position will keep pressure off your neck and shoulders. It's the proper posture for your mid to upper spine.

After doing these workouts, your body should involuntarily start to squeeze the bones on its own. This is your DNA at work. You may notice yourself start to walk funny, maybe like a baby. Your butt will stick out pretty good. Your adductors will stretch out, slightly separating the fronts of your legs. Your posture will become flawless. That's your whole goal here, to make that curve bigger.

Walk according to the position your underdeveloped muscles want to be in. Don't be so fast to walk. Take shorter strides, and relax your adductors as you're walking. You should find yourself walking more with the back of your hip bone pushed up into your lower back, and your legs sucked up into their socket better. Your butt should stick out like a baby.

Hamstring

The hamstring is actually responsible for 3 movements, but I have found the only one that might need addressing is the curling motion, bending at the knees. I have tried to work the hamstring by doing a type of squat that doesn't utilize the thigh muscles but that just pushed against my posture and didn't seem to have any real benefit any way. The core muscles really seem to comprise the entire problem of hip misalignment. But, if your situation is different and you discover you do need to work your hamstrings a little, I recommend sticking to leg curls on a machine. Any machine will do, except the ones where you have to lay on your stomach.

Traps

People like to work the chest to make it look good and huge, but fail to realize that they are putting unruly pressure on the shoulders and neck. Office workers may be putting similar stress on their neck and shoulders sitting at a computer all day. To check this pressure, do the following:

Stand or sit holding a pair of dumbbells. Flex ONLY the trap muscles, bringing your shoulders straight up. You may hear some cracks or pops as your shoulder is brought back into its socket better.

Rear Deltoids

You can work this muscle in a variety of ways. There are free weights, like dumbbells, or machines and pulleys. I like to use free weights while lying on a bench. That way you have resistance through the full range of motion.

Lie on a bench, face down, with a dumbbell in each hand. You won't have to use very heavy dumbbells, as your chest compression on the bench will already provide some resistance. Letting your arms hang loosely, squeeze only the rear deltoid muscles. Bring them all the way up as far as you can, then slowly bring the back down with control.

Rotator Cuff

This is probably one of the muscles least affected in chronic shoulder pain, but still can cause a problem none-the-less. To work this muscle, all you have to do is bend your arm at the elbow and rotate your forearm back, until it's in line with your body. If this muscle is underdeveloped, you should feel a slight crunching sound in the base of your neck and shoulder area, where the muscle connects to the spine. It's a good crunching sound. Your vertebrae are getting pulled back in alignment.

Inner Triceps

One way to strengthen the inner triceps would be to use dumbbells to do overhead triceps extensions. You would just sit on a bench, or even just stand, hold a dumbbell above your head with your arm extended, and bend your arm to lower the dumbbell toward your shoulder. The more effective way to strengthen this muscle would be to do dips. You would just prop yourself up between two parallel bars, then lower and raise yourself using just the triceps (to the best of your ability). Try not to incorporate the front deltoids. If this kind of dip is too difficult, you could do as assisted dip with a machine at the gym.

End of exercise list.

In the world of muscle building, we call doing multiple exercises at once like this circuit training. It's a great workout and replaces cardio exercises like running and biking. I don't recommend ever doing traditional cardio exercises again, if you want to maintain your posture and hip, knee, and ankle alignments. If you want to do continual movement for 5 to 10 minutes or longer, you can simply do hundreds of reps of any of the above exercises, with light weights – your new cardio.

To build muscle mass and strength, a very effective mode of weight training is tri sets. Tri sets are 3 sets using no more weight than you can lift 5, 10, and 20 times per set, respectively. Lifting a weight you can lift only five times shreds your large twitch muscles and builds their strength. Lifting a weight you can lift no more than 8-10 times further fatigues the large twitch muscle for endurance. Lifting a weight you can lift no more than 20 times works the small, fast twitch muscles. I built almost 20 pounds of muscle using this technique (unfortunately that was when I worked out improperly, and ended up being a major contributor to my muscle imbalances!). Careful with tri sets in the core. I discovered it's difficult to maintain good form when using heavy weights.

Another way to build and tighten muscle is to do endurance lifts. This is where you'll do 50 – 100 reps of a certain motion. Keep flexing until you give out - which is called "failure", in weightlifting terms. If you can do more than 100 reps, add weight. If you can't do 50 reps, reduce the weight. After all, endurance is probably one of the reasons you're suffering from chronic structural problems –thousands upon thousands of repetitions in those overdeveloped muscles. This technique will really tighten the underdeveloped muscles and neutralize the antagonistic muscles. I've found it has different benefits than doing tri sets. I recommend doing both types of lifting (on different days of course) for maximum, and quickest, results.

An effective technique to working out is to take your time. Hold your lifts at the peak for a second or two, then release. When you're releasing, don't simply relax, or give out. Take a couple seconds to let the weight down, controlled. Experts say that the decline is just as important as the lift. It appears they're right. Lifts can get pretty difficult when you hold for a second or two and release slowly. This means better gains in strength.

You'll see results during and immediately after your first workout. The problem is that a casual walk or any type of manual labor will probably throw your hip right back out of alignment. Daily activities will push that hip and spine back out of alignment frequently. If you have to bend over and lift heavier objects, bend at the knees. It's the least stressful bent over position on your hip. It will probably take at least 2 months to see longer lasting, hopefully permanent, results. I still have slight problems keeping my hip where it belongs, but it's 10 times better than it used to be. Being the upright species really takes its toll on our body. Recovery will take serious work, but it's achievable.

Also, remember that you can flex any muscle you want, any time you want. If you feel a bone slip or something, go ahead and flex muscles until you find the problem. You've made a correction if you hear a pop or crack. Over time, you'll be able to figure out exactly what muscle you need to flex to correct a bone misalignment. Be sure and flex really hard because the muscles imbalances are probably pretty severe. It will take some serious effort to pull against those overly tight back, leg, and perhaps chest muscles.

Keep in mind that just because you do an exercise one day doesn't mean your hip will stay in that position the rest of the day. The daily activity and the years of stress these underdeveloped muscles have been under will continue to be a drag on your hip and spine for some time. It's like taking two steps forward and one step back. But after each successive workout, the likelihood of going all the way back to "square one" diminishes. Your goal is to build enough muscle to where this new muscle can neutralize the stress of their overdeveloped, antagonistic counterparts.

By no means is the above an exhaustive list of exercises. Be creative! There probably are lifts I haven't discovered yet.

Especially make sure *each lift is done so that you cannot move the weight any further*. Follow through. Don't be wimpy! Lift like you mean it. Crush those overdeveloped muscles. This is crucial to making every muscle fiber of any muscle group strong and also to make it look good all around.

Your joints will probably sound like a bowl of Rice Krispies when you flex these weaker core muscles – lots of snaps, cracks, and pops. This may happen throughout the day, too. It's a good thing. That's the alignment being fixed. I believe my ex-chiropractor told me it's a pocket of air leaving or entering the joint.

Walking Posture
After working these core muscles and getting up off the chair, you should naturally walk around with your legs back, butt back, upper body pulled back, back arched and taller, and walking slow and awkward. That's exactly where you want to be. That means you're doing it right. You should also notice some benefits in biological functions around the hip.

Do NOT kick so hard to walk forward. You are not going to crunch to walk forward any more. Relax your adductors as best you can, and let your upper body walk taller – shoulders up and back, and chest out. Do not slouch. Allow yourself to walk tall. If your upper body becomes disinclined to walking tall, you need to reset your core. Walking with a good posture should be natural.

Also - if you're not ambidextrous - after strengthening these formerly neglected muscles in your core, your mid section may want to be a little crooked when you stand and walk around. It may even be inclined to twist a little, pushing your dominant hip forward and stretching out that dominant low back muscle. That's normal and good. Yes, it's awkward, but this is your body automatically trying to neutralize the stress your overdeveloped muscles are putting on the hip. It's the muscles' new natural positioning to neutralize strength from the overdeveloped muscles. It's pretty much your dominant leg being sucked back up into its socket better. It'll have to be maintained even in the sitting and sleeping postures. Hey, whatever works.

Remember how I told you that your dominant oblique could be stretched out, with your non dominant oblique being accommodated/shortened? This crooked positioning is your body automatically trying to shorten the dominant oblique and lengthen the non dominant oblique, neutralizing the strength of your overdeveloped muscles in the back and legs. It should feel real good when this starts to occur. It may look funny, but it's well worth the relief. When you're walking right, your upper body will want to lean back as well. This emphasizes the curves in your spine. Being upright is the least stressful position on the hip and spine (outside the womb that is).

Remember the GI Joe analogy? When you're doing this workout program you should feel the back of your hip kind of jam up into your lower back and stretch it out back there. This will make your butt stick back and pull your upper body back. This is your hip being pulled back up into your mid section. Tighten the neglected muscles and the hip will get sucked back up into its socket; and the posture will return to its natural, curvy position. That curve only exists because of the position of your hip bone. Try to keep this position 24/7.

Your body will naturally want to shift the back of your hip up into your lower back and suck your mid section down into your hip socket. You will usually have to consciously allow it to do so while you're walking around, if you want to fully resist structural problems and stretch those leg and back muscles back out. This will help arch your lower spine back real good. Like I told you in the correct postures section earlier, there's a certain position you have to put your hip. It will probably take some practice. When you've hit or come close to this posture in any of the 3 positions (sleeping, sitting, walking/standing), you're pretty much there. At this point, you are light years ahead of your former posture.

Supplements

Keep in mind, like anything, the more you invest, the faster and better you will achieve results. Supplements for muscle building will go a long way in your recovery from chronic pain and digestive problems. The starter supplement would be protein. More optional (but still effective) supplements would be nitric oxide boosters, creatine, natural growth hormone enhancement supplements, testosterone boosters and more.

The building blocks for muscle are amino acids. Amino acids are the peptide chains that complete proteins consist of. Quality protein and a lot of it is essential for muscle strength and recovery. Most people on the typical western diet are deficient in protein. It is very difficult to get quality protein and other important nutrients, like MSM (methylsulfonylmethane) and enzymes, in substantial, life sustaining amounts, from our overcooked diet. In "The Diet and Nutrition Super Manual: How to Truly Eat Clean, Lose Fat and Build Muscle Fast Without Exercise", I prove how this deficiency can keep people from losing weight, even and especially those who exercise. Quality protein builds lean muscle to burn fat more effectively. In nearly every case I've ever seen, it's worked like that. It is virtually impossible to build lean muscle without ample quality protein in your diet. It will also help you stay fuller, longer; cut cravings; improve hair, focus and energy levels, etc. If you're serious about building muscle to reverse the stress caused by overdeveloped muscles, protein supplementation is not optional.

The market has been churning out some great supplements in recent years:

- Prime Muscle Pill - very potent muscle builder, possibly a testosterone boosting supplement. Its main ingredient is some kind of plant extract, so it's all natural and hypo-allergenic.

- Powerfull or Royal Velvet: all natural growth hormone enhancers. Like muscle on demand. Hypo-allergenic.

- Nitric Oxide boosters - expand blood vessels, allowing for more nutrient absorption. Very effective for strength and endurance. I use anything with a good blend of L-arginine, or L-citrulline, and beta alanine.

- Creatine - CE2 is creatine in a pill. Cellmass is another solid product.

- Just about any whey protein and protein blend – most have many ingredients added to repair and grow muscle. But if you're a health fanatic like me (and you're allergic to traditional dairy), then your best bet for clean protein is whey protein made from grass fed cows. Grass fed bovine protein is more nutrient dense and has less inflammatory omega-6 fat than corn and grain fed cows.

Another whey protein alternative is goat whey. There are also veggie proteins, like rice, hemp, pea, etc. Each of these is unique, but not as effective at building muscle (and keeping your hair thick) as whey.

All these supplements are powerful and effective by themselves, but combining them will yield steroid-like results so your bones can stay in alignment better. Using multiple performance supplements at once is called "stacking". They're usually taken before workouts, so they're classified as "preworkout" supplements. Variations of these products and new products from their competitors arrive on the market just about daily. See my Supplement Corner page at letmybodygo.com for quick access to some of these supplements.

It's not a supplement, but there's a gel you can apply topically to a muscle to make it to loosen up. It's called Bio-freeze. I've tried it a few times and it works like magic. I've used it on the low back muscle and hip flexor. It really does loosen up over developed muscles. But it's certainly not a replacement for muscle strengthening.

Nutrition

While many people believe nutrition plays the primary or only role in chronic pain and digestive problems, it's actually not the primary factor. It does play a role, but it's not nearly as much of a factor as muscle imbalances. I know this, not only from my own experience, but watching others. I watch people who have to rely on supplements to keep inflammation away. As long they take their supplement, the pain stays away. But if they stop taking their supplement, the pain returns. This is because those nutrients are only dealing with a symptom of the pain, not the core problem. It may work to keep the pain away, but who wants to have to be dependent on costly supplements?

Nutrition is important in that it will help to strengthen and rebuild your body as you restore your posture. It helps in that it will strengthen your body at the cellular/DNA level. When you can feed your DNA the nutrients it needs to remain intact longer, you can make your body as a whole stay tighter, longer, and not have to be dependent so much on the ab lounge. Nutrition helps you flex stronger when you go to strengthen the long neglected muscles, and keep them strong when you aren't flexing. This helps you better pull against the stronger antagonist muscles and take the stress off the nerves, bones and connective tissue stuck in the middle.

While protein may be the most important nutrient in strengthening your muscles to reverse severe muscle imbalances, there are others that are still very important, like carbohydrates and hydrogen. Carbs actually work with protein to build and maintain muscle, and are the best source for muscle and mental energy. Carbs are critical for workouts and muscle mass retention. Hydrogen actually comes from carbs (carboHYDRates?). Hydrogen is about the most critical nutrient in the food supply. Hydrogen is energy. It is also an antioxidant, and it's necessary for DNA health. The double helix strands that compose your DNA are held together by hydrogen bonds. Your connective tissue - basically your last line of defense against chronic pain - is comprised of hydrogen. So basically, a deficiency of hydrogen results in the breakdown of your body at the cellular level. Hydrogen is essentially the cushioning around your body that helps to prevent chronic pain and a slew of other conditions. Other nutrients, like electrolytes, vitamins and minerals support carb and protein synthesis and utilization, so you really must consume nutrient dense foods to aid in your recovery.

For a complete breakdown of the importance of hydrogen, the best sources, and all other nutrients, and exactly how food effects your body, read my book, "The Diet and Nutrition Super Manual". This book shows you exactly what goes into weight control, exactly why obesity is so prevalent in our society, and how to stay slim down to your muscle. This book details the 7 factors that compose perfect health, great immunity, great energy levels, exposes all the common weight control myths, and so on. It's a must if you expect to live strong and live long, physically and mentally.

Stretching
One last technique that may prove to add more results to your recovery is stretching. Stretching the overdeveloped muscles will take some pressure off the joints they're attached to, and further reduce recovery time. It's tough to stretch the back muscles without wrecking posture. The renewed position of your hip will do that for you. Some muscle groups you can stretch are the ones in the front of your legs – the adductors, flexors and thighs. You could sit on the floor with your legs crossed and push your knees close to the floor. Some times I lay on my bed in a similar position with my legs crossed. Flex the pelvis and abdomen, or dominant oblique, while stretching, to suck the hip tight into its socket and further stretch the overdeveloped muscles. When you get up to walk, you may have a whole new stride. It should feel pretty good.

Like just about anything in life, practice makes perfect. It is going to take a conscious effort to avoid the activities and positions that strain your underdeveloped core, or any other muscles. It will probably take some trial and error. The hip is very complex. Certain muscles loosen easily, and it's not always easy to tell which ones. I'll admit, I still screw up, and probably always will. To this day, I'm still restoring my bones. One bad workout can make all my progress come to a screeching halt. Fortunately, screwing up rarely entails much pain. The severe pain is the first to go in this recovery process, and takes a lot to come back. The discomfort may hang around. You don't have to go through as much of the trial and error as I did. You now have the blueprints neatly outlined for you. Consider me your guinea pig for all these techniques.

You're now equipped to conquer structural problems due to muscle imbalances instantly, possibly within day or weeks. You really can restore your bones and biological functions back to the positions they were born in.

Walk slower. Allow the back of your hip to naturally slide up into its socket, stick your butt back, and allow for a big arch to your lower spine. It's all about body mechanics.

The correct postures and muscle balances will keep much pressure off of the vertebrae. This makes it more difficult for them to slip out of alignment. In essence, the correct postures and muscle balances keep you pain free, comfortable, off of expensive drugs, and out of costly doctor and chiropractor offices. You'll see vast improvements!

And don't be surprised if you start experiencing weight loss from all the exercise, fidgeting, and renewed digestive system (I'm sure you're bummed, huh?).

If this is your first time reading this book through, I suggest you go back and read it again. Knowing what you know now may help you get an even better grasp on the big picture and your specific problems as you read it all again. There may a thing or two you didn't totally understand or see which will become clearer by reading it again.

Questions, comments, concerns? Send me an email – bodymechanic@letmybodygo.com. I love hearing from people I've helped. I'm all about results. If you are having a structural problem and somehow nothing in this e-book helps it, I would like to know about it. I may even be able to help.

Social Media

You can stay in tune with the latest in greatest in health and wellness and follow me on social media as I release all my tips, tools, secrets and videos. Share this information with everyone you think will benefit from it. And please tell others about your results and opinion of this book, and rate and review it where you bought it. Help the world free itself from its bondage to poor health by sharing this life changing information.

Facebook: www.facebook.com/letmybodygo and click the "Like" button at the top to follow.

Youtube: www.youtube.com/letmybodygo

Twitter: @bodymechanic7

Blog and resources: www.letmybodygo.com

References

1. http://news.bbc.co.uk/1/hi/health/6058008.stm

2. http://orthopedics.about.com/gi/dynamic/offsite.htm?zi=1/XJ&sdn=orthopedics&cdn=health&tm=17&gps=267_49_1020_592&f=00&su=p284.9.336.ip_p736.3.336.ip_&tt=2&bt=0&bts=0&zu=http%3A//orthoinfo.aaos.org/fact/thr_report.cfm%3FThread_ID%3D93%26topcategory%3DAbout%2520Orthopaedics

http://cenkchiro.com/treatments/core-stabilization/

More Health and Wellness Books

If you want more truth in health and wellness, get my other books:

"The Diet and Nutrition Super Manual: How to Truly Eat Clean, Lose Fat and Build Muscle Without Exercise"

"Fire Your Doctor: How to Not Get Sick. Ever. Seriously."

"How I Cured My Chronic Acne: How to Get Rid of Blackheads, Pimples and Zits With a Nutritional Approach"

And if you graciously write a review of this book where you bought it, I will GIVE you any other book I've written, your choice. Same offer goes for all those other books. That's right, you can get the health secrets of the universe - all my books - for free, just for spending two minutes typing a few sentences. Just shoot me an email at info@letmybodygo.com with the link to your review and I'll reply with the pdf file. It's that simple. I look forward to hearing from you!

There's more good news. You can actually earn money referring my powerful books to your network of friends, family and associates. And it's incredibly quick and easy to set up.

My books have high conversion rates and people fall in love with them. Plus, the health and wellness industry is booming and growing. The average person cares about their health, wants to eat healthy, avoid pain, live as long as possible, not get sick and save money on ineffective products, foods and medical expenses. People want health and wealth security, and my books cover all these areas. I am a health, money and efficiency fanatic (I actually have a degree in accounting). I have done some amazing things with my health and pocketbook. I've saved and transformed my health in many ways, improved my quality of life and saved a ton of money in the process. I will never have to rely on the medical establishment. I am my own doctor. And I documented virtually the entire adventure in my books. It's things like this people crave. I've helped many people overcome sever health problems, and many people have run to me for help with their health because they know I know what I'm doing. People want the truth, especially when it comes to health and wellness.

Promoting other people's products on the internet is 100% profit (unless you choose to spend $ on marketing). No overhead. No production costs. No delivery. No collections. That's passive, easy income. That's efficiency, and that's power. All you need to do is get the message out and generate some buzz via social media, videos, articles, whatever. Your results will sell. You can post your results and fascination from my books on some forums. Testimonials, results and excitement sell big time. When I first got started marketing this book, I made around 5 - 10 responses to posts on some chronic pain forums that didn't look like spam. I just said something like 'the problem is muscles imbalances... I got relief from a book on Amazon. Just search "[How I Cured...]"'. It was all true, offered the real solution to the poster's problem, and within just a few months those posts were earning me $6-20 per month. That's not much at all, but it's free money, pure profit, it was just a start for one book in digital form only at the time; and as long as those forums exist, I'll be making money from those brief and free posts. Imagine doing that with all my books in digital and hard copy formats. Could you use an extra $50, $75, $100 or more per month?

Some wealth guru teaches that everyone should have 21 lines of income. I agree wholeheartedly. What's better - one big income that never grows, or multiple small to large lines of income that grow perpetually? That's a no brainer. And that's security.

You typically don't even have to cultivate lines of income like this, just "set it and forget it" - residual income. You could make some videos on Youtube with your results and impression from my books. You could do some Twitter searches for keywords and posts containing problems my books will solve and reply to the list of posts that show up. You can reply to people's posts on forums. You can even generate a brief report detailing your recovery from chronic pain, publish it yourself on sites like Amazon Kindle or Draft 2 Digital, or post it wherever you can upload a file, slap a $0 price tag on it for maximum traffic, and plug my other books containing your affiliate links to make money on them. Do stuff like that, generate some buzz and you are "off to the races". Buzz and excitement are contagious, and contagious = money. By the way, if you choose to publish your report or ebook on Amazon Kindle, you must publish it somewhere else that allows you to price the product at $0. Then you must show the sales page to Amazon support and ask them to match the price. Otherwise, you will only be able to do free book promotions on Kindle for 5 days, every 90 days.

To get started as an Amazon affiliate, you simply sign up for an account at Amazon Associates. Then search their product search engine on the Associates Central/home page to automatically generate your affiliate links. Take those links and post them with your results and excitement on your social media, videos, digital signatures and anywhere else you think people can benefit from them. You can get paper checks or direct deposit your commissions and automate the entire process.

It probably won't start out as much income initially, depending on the size of your networks and how many posts you make. But over time, your lines of income will grow. They have for me. As long as the population and internet grow, your seeds will grow. And "the sky is the limit" with the internet. Plus, the more seeds you sow, the more you reap.

Some slicksters game the system and earn a bunch of money publishing hundreds of low quality books that each make small amounts of money. I have a bunch of high quality books you can promote, they're optimized for maximum conversion rate, and I always have more in the works. So stay tuned to my social media for new releases so you can read them, get results and get your affiliate links.

We all refer and brag about our solutions and results to our human network. Why not earn money for it, in your sleep? It would be silly not to.

The harvest is immense and the laborers are few. The truth needs a big work force to help the world relieve some of the most debilitating conditions we face. There is so much information out there but none of it is as accurate, concise, and condensed as my books. Promote that fact. Bash the ineffective competition. It's true and it sells. But you must sow the seeds sooner rather than later. Lines of income like this typically grow, but it takes time. Enlist at Amazon Associates today and earn some easy money!